PESCATERIAN DIABETIC DIET COOKBOOK FOR SENIORS

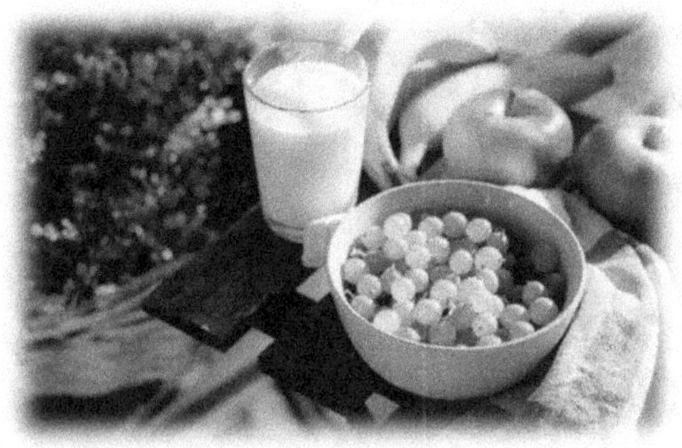

Healthy plant based and seafood recipes to manage Diabetes for seniors

DR.LINDA MCDANIEL

TABLE OF CONTENT

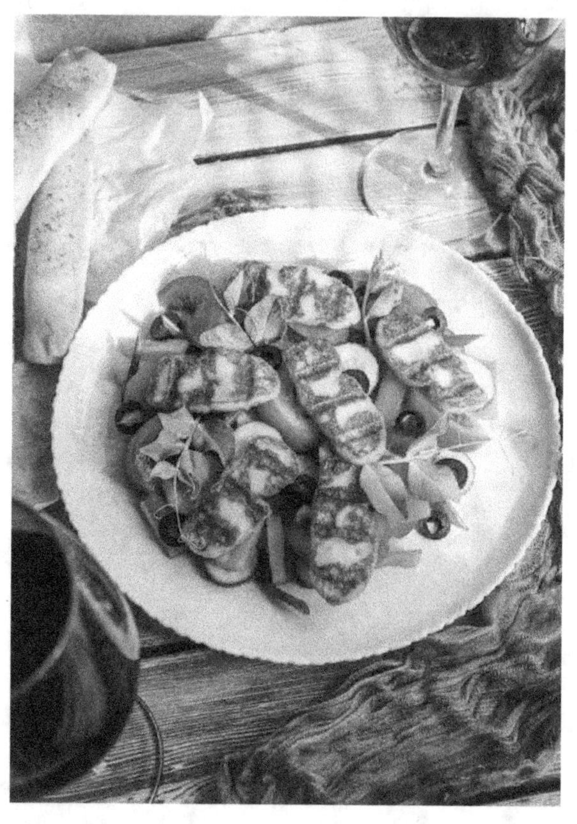

INTRODUCTION

Welcome to the Pescaterian Diet Cookbook for Seniors: Nutritious and Flavorful Anti-inflammatory Recipes to Naturally Combat and Enhance Good Health. As a seasoned nutritionist with years of experience, I am thrilled to present this comprehensive guide tailored specifically for seniors navigating the complexities of managing diabetes through dietary choices.

Living with diabetes presents unique challenges, particularly as we age. It necessitates a thoughtful approach to nutrition—one that prioritizes both health and enjoyment. In this cookbook, you will find a wealth of recipes meticulously crafted to support your journey towards optimal well-being.

The pescatarian diet, centered around plant-based foods with the inclusion of fish and seafood, offers a myriad of health benefits, particularly for those managing diabetes.

By emphasizing nutrient-rich ingredients and harnessing the power of anti-inflammatory foods, each recipe within these pages is designed not only to tantalize your taste buds but also to promote wellness from within.

Through my years of practice, I have witnessed firsthand the transformative impact that dietary modifications can have on overall health. By adopting a pescatarian approach and incorporating anti-inflammatory ingredients, we can harness the healing potential of food to combat inflammation, manage blood sugar levels, and cultivate vitality.

Within this cookbook, you will embark on a culinary journey brimming with vibrant flavors, nourishing ingredients, and healthful indulgences. From hearty mains to delightful desserts, each recipe is thoughtfully curated to strike the perfect balance between deliciousness and nutrition.

Whether you are new to the pescatarian lifestyle or a seasoned advocate, whether you are seeking inspiration for weeknight dinners or special occasions, this cookbook is your trusted companion on the path to wellness. Together, let us savor the joys of wholesome eating and celebrate the transformative power of food as medicine.

Here's to embracing vibrant health, one delicious bite at a time.

With warmest regards,

Dr. Linda McDaniel

Nutritionist and Author

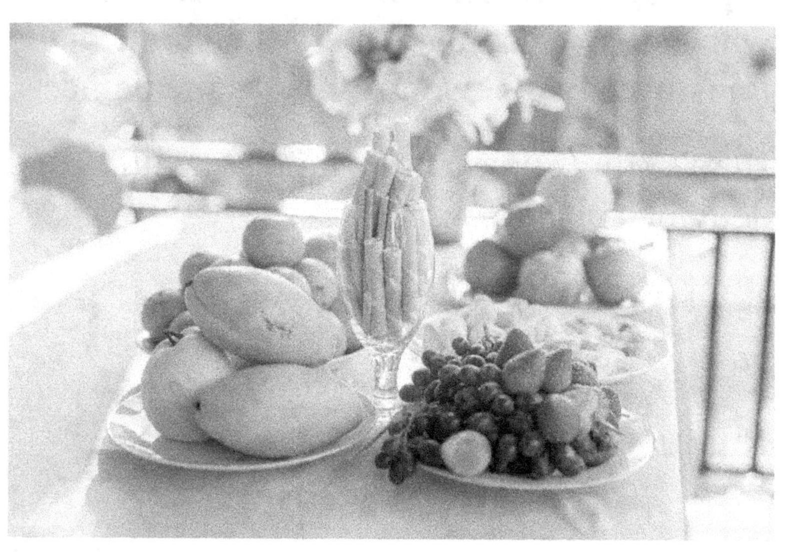

CHAPTER 1

Understanding Diabetes: Types, Causes, Symptoms, and Preventive Measures

Diabetes mellitus, commonly referred to as diabetes, is a chronic metabolic disorder characterized by elevated blood sugar levels over a prolonged period. This condition arises due to either insufficient production of insulin—a hormone responsible for regulating blood sugar—or the body's ineffective use of the insulin it produces. Diabetes poses significant health risks if left unmanaged, contributing to various complications affecting multiple organ systems. In this comprehensive exploration, we delve into the types, causes, symptoms, and preventive measures for diabetes.

Types of Diabetes:

1. **Type 1 Diabetes:** Also known as insulin-dependent diabetes mellitus (IDDM),

   Type 1 diabetes typically develops during childhood or adolescence but can occur at any age. It results from the immune system mistakenly attacking and destroying the insulin-producing beta cells in the pancreas. Individuals with Type 1 diabetes require lifelong insulin therapy to manage their blood sugar levels.

2. **Type 2 Diabetes:** Formerly referred to as non-insulin-dependent diabetes mellitus (NIDDM), Type 2 diabetes is the most prevalent form, comprising approximately 90% of all diabetes cases worldwide. It typically manifests in adulthood, although the prevalence among younger individuals, including adolescents and children,

is increasing. Type 2 diabetes develops when the body becomes resistant to insulin or fails to produce enough insulin to meet its needs. Lifestyle factors, such as poor dietary habits, sedentary lifestyle, and obesity, significantly contribute to the development of Type 2 diabetes.

3. **Gestational Diabetes:** Gestational diabetes mellitus (GDM) occurs during pregnancy when hormonal changes lead to insulin resistance. While it often resolves after childbirth, women with gestational diabetes have an increased risk of developing Type 2 diabetes later in life. Proper management during pregnancy is essential to minimize risks to both the mother and the baby.

Causes of Diabetes:

The causes of diabetes vary depending on the type but often involve a combination of genetic, environmental, and lifestyle factors.

In Type 1 diabetes, an autoimmune response triggers the destruction of pancreatic beta cells, leading to insulin deficiency. While the exact cause remains unclear, genetic predisposition and environmental triggers, such as viral infections, are believed to play a role.

Type 2 diabetes primarily develops due to insulin resistance—a condition in which the body's cells become less responsive to insulin—or inadequate insulin production by the pancreas. Obesity, physical inactivity, unhealthy dietary habits, and genetic factors contribute to the development of insulin resistance and Type 2 diabetes. Gestational diabetes arises from hormonal changes during pregnancy, leading to elevated blood sugar levels.

Symptoms of Diabetes:

The symptoms of diabetes vary in severity and may develop gradually or suddenly, depending on the type and individual factors. Common symptoms include:

- **Frequent urination (polyuria):** Excessive sugar in the blood leads to increased urine production, causing frequent urination.

- **Excessive thirst (polydipsia):** Dehydration resulting from frequent urination triggers increased thirst.

- **Unexplained weight loss:** Despite increased appetite, individuals may experience weight loss due to the body's inability to effectively utilize glucose for energy.

- **Fatigue:** Insufficient glucose uptake by cells leads to fatigue and weakness.

- **Blurred vision:** High blood sugar levels can affect the eye's lens, leading to blurred vision or other vision problems.

- **Slow wound healing:** Diabetes impairs the body's ability to heal wounds and increases the risk of infections.

- **Numbness or tingling in extremities:** Peripheral neuropathy, a common complication of diabetes,

  causes numbness, tingling, or pain in the hands and feet.

- **Frequent infections:** Elevated blood sugar levels weaken the immune system, increasing the risk of infections, particularly in the urinary tract, skin, and gums.

Preventive Measures for Diabetes:

While certain risk factors for diabetes, such as genetic predisposition, cannot be modified, adopting a healthy lifestyle can significantly reduce the risk of developing Type 2 diabetes and help manage Type 1 diabetes effectively. Key preventive measures include:

1. **Healthy Diet:** Emphasize a balanced diet rich in fruits, vegetables, whole grains, lean proteins, and healthy fats. Limit intake of refined carbohydrates,

sugary foods, and beverages to prevent blood sugar spikes.

2. **Regular Physical Activity:** Engage in regular exercise, such as brisk walking, cycling, swimming, or strength training, to improve insulin sensitivity, lower blood sugar levels, and maintain a healthy weight.

3. **Weight Management:** Maintain a healthy body weight through a combination of dietary modifications and regular exercise. Even modest weight loss can significantly reduce the risk of developing Type 2 diabetes.

4. **Monitoring Blood Sugar Levels:** Individuals with diabetes should monitor their blood sugar levels regularly using glucometers and adhere to their prescribed treatment plan, including insulin therapy or oral medications.

5. **Stress Management:** Practice stress-reducing techniques, such as mindfulness meditation, deep breathing exercises, or yoga,

    to minimize the impact of stress hormones on blood sugar levels.

6. **Avoidance of Smoking and Excessive Alcohol Consumption:** Smoking and excessive alcohol intake can worsen insulin resistance and increase the risk of cardiovascular complications associated with diabetes. Quit smoking and limit alcohol consumption to reduce these risks.

7. **Regular Medical Check-ups:** Schedule regular check-ups with healthcare providers to monitor blood sugar levels, assess overall health, and address any emerging complications or concerns promptly.

CHAPTER 2

Optimizing Health with a Diabetes Pescatarian Diet

A pescatarian diet, rich in plant-based foods and supplemented with fish and seafood, offers seniors managing diabetes a delicious and nutritious approach to achieving optimum health. By focusing on nutrient-dense ingredients and mindful meal planning, seniors can effectively manage blood sugar levels, reduce inflammation, and support overall well-being. Here's a guide to the foods to eat and avoid for seniors following a diabetes pescatarian diet:

Foods to Eat:

1. **Vegetables:** Load up on non-starchy vegetables such as leafy greens, broccoli, cauliflower, bell peppers, and Brussels sprouts. These vegetables are low in calories and carbohydrates

while being packed with essential vitamins, minerals, and fiber,

which help regulate blood sugar levels and promote digestive health.

2. **Fruits:** Opt for low-glycemic fruits like berries (strawberries, blueberries, raspberries), apples, pears, and citrus fruits. These fruits are rich in antioxidants, fiber, and vitamins, providing sweetness without causing significant spikes in blood sugar levels.

3. **Whole Grains:** Choose whole grains such as quinoa, brown rice, barley, oats, and whole wheat products over refined grains. Whole grains are high in fiber, which slows down the absorption of sugar into the bloodstream, helping to stabilize blood sugar levels and promote satiety.

4. **Legumes:** Incorporate legumes like lentils, chickpeas, black beans, and kidney beans into your meals.

Legumes are excellent sources of plant-based protein, fiber,

and complex carbohydrates, which aid in blood sugar control and promote heart health.

5. **Fatty Fish:** Include fatty fish such as salmon, mackerel, sardines, and trout in your diet regularly. These fish are rich in omega-3 fatty acids, which have anti-inflammatory properties and support cardiovascular health. Aim for at least two servings of fatty fish per week.

6. **Nuts and Seeds:** Snack on a variety of nuts and seeds, including almonds, walnuts, chia seeds, and flaxseeds. These nutrient-dense snacks are rich in healthy fats, protein, and fiber, making them excellent choices for blood sugar management and satiety.

7. **Healthy Fats:** Incorporate sources of healthy fats such as olive oil, avocado,

and coconut oil into your cooking and salads.

These fats help improve insulin sensitivity, reduce inflammation, and support brain health.

8. **Dairy Alternatives:** Choose unsweetened dairy alternatives like almond milk, soy milk, or coconut yogurt. These options provide calcium and protein without the added sugars found in traditional dairy products.

Foods to Avoid:

1. **Processed Foods:** Minimize consumption of processed foods, including sugary snacks, baked goods, processed meats, and convenience foods. These foods are often high in refined carbohydrates, unhealthy fats, and added sugars, which can lead to blood sugar spikes and inflammation.

2. **Sugary Beverages:** Avoid sugary drinks such as soda, fruit juices, and sweetened teas, as they contribute to rapid increases in blood sugar levels. Opt for water, herbal teas,

   or infused water with lemon or cucumber for hydration.

3. **Highly Processed Grains:** Limit intake of highly processed grains like white bread, white rice, and pasta, which lack fiber and nutrients. Instead, choose whole grain alternatives for better blood sugar control and overall health.

4. **Saturated and Trans Fats:** Reduce consumption of foods high in saturated and trans fats, such as fried foods, fatty cuts of meat, and full-fat dairy products. These fats can increase inflammation and raise the risk of heart disease.

5. **Salty Foods:** Cut back on foods high in sodium, such as processed snacks,

canned soups, and salty condiments. Excessive sodium intake can contribute to high blood pressure and increase the risk of cardiovascular complications.

6. **Sweetened Condiments:** Avoid condiments and sauces containing added sugars, such as ketchup, barbecue sauce, and sweet chili sauce. Opt for homemade or low-sugar alternatives to control sugar intake.

By following a diabetes pescatarian diet rich in nutrient-dense whole foods and mindful eating habits, seniors can effectively manage their blood sugar levels, reduce inflammation, and support overall health and well-being. Embrace the abundance of delicious and wholesome ingredients available and savor the journey to optimum health.

CHAPTER 3

Step by step dietary approach

Following a diabetic pescatarian diet for seniors involves careful planning and thoughtful food choices to manage blood sugar levels effectively while supporting overall health. Here's a step-by-step guide on how seniors can navigate this dietary approach:

1. Consult with a Healthcare Professional: Before making any significant changes to your diet, consult with a registered dietitian or healthcare provider specializing in diabetes management. They can provide personalized recommendations based on your health status, medication regimen, and individual dietary needs.

2. Understand Dietary Guidelines: Familiarize yourself with dietary guidelines for managing diabetes and adopting a pescatarian lifestyle.

Focus on consuming a variety of nutrient-dense foods while controlling portion sizes and monitoring carbohydrate intake to maintain stable blood sugar levels.

3. Plan Balanced Meals: Plan well-balanced meals that incorporate a combination of lean proteins, healthy fats, fiber-rich carbohydrates, and plenty of non-starchy vegetables. Aim to fill half of your plate with vegetables, one-quarter with protein-rich foods, and one-quarter with whole grains or legumes.

4. Choose Quality Protein Sources: Include a variety of fish and seafood in your diet to meet protein needs while minimizing saturated fat intake. Opt for fatty fish rich in omega-3 fatty acids, such as salmon, mackerel, and sardines, which have anti-inflammatory properties and support heart health.

5. Emphasize Plant-Based Foods: Prioritize plant-based foods such as fruits, vegetables, whole grains, legumes, nuts, and seeds. These foods are rich in fiber, vitamins, minerals, and antioxidants, which promote satiety, regulate blood sugar levels, and reduce the risk of chronic diseases.

6. Control Carbohydrate Intake: Monitor carbohydrate intake and focus on choosing high-fiber, low-glycemic options to minimize blood sugar spikes. Include whole grains like quinoa, brown rice, and barley, as well as legumes like lentils and chickpeas, which provide sustained energy without causing rapid fluctuations in blood glucose levels.

7. Limit Added Sugars and Processed Foods: Avoid or minimize consumption of sugary snacks, desserts, and processed foods, which can contribute to elevated blood sugar levels and inflammation. Opt for whole, minimally processed foods whenever possible and sweeten foods naturally with fruit or small amounts of honey or maple syrup.

8. Monitor Portion Sizes: Pay attention to portion sizes to avoid overeating and maintain a healthy weight. Use measuring cups, food scales, or visual cues to gauge appropriate serving sizes of different food groups, especially carbohydrate-rich foods like grains and fruits.

9. Stay Hydrated: Drink plenty of water throughout the day to stay hydrated and support optimal health. Limit consumption of sugary beverages and opt for calorie-free options like water, herbal teas, or infused water with fresh fruits and herbs.

10. Monitor Blood Sugar Levels: Regularly monitor blood sugar levels using a glucometer as recommended by your healthcare provider. Keep track of your dietary choices, physical activity levels, and medication regimen to identify patterns and make necessary adjustments to your diabetes management plan.

11. Be Mindful of Sodium Intake: Limit intake of high-sodium foods like processed snacks, canned soups, and salty condiments to support heart health and reduce the risk of hypertension. Choose low-sodium alternatives or flavor foods with herbs, spices, and citrus juices instead.

12. Practice Mindful Eating: Practice mindful eating by paying attention to hunger and fullness cues, savoring each bite, and eating slowly to prevent overeating. Focus on enjoying meals in a relaxed environment free from distractions, such as television or electronic devices.

By following these guidelines and making informed dietary choices, seniors can effectively manage diabetes while enjoying a varied and delicious pescatarian diet that promotes overall health and well-being.

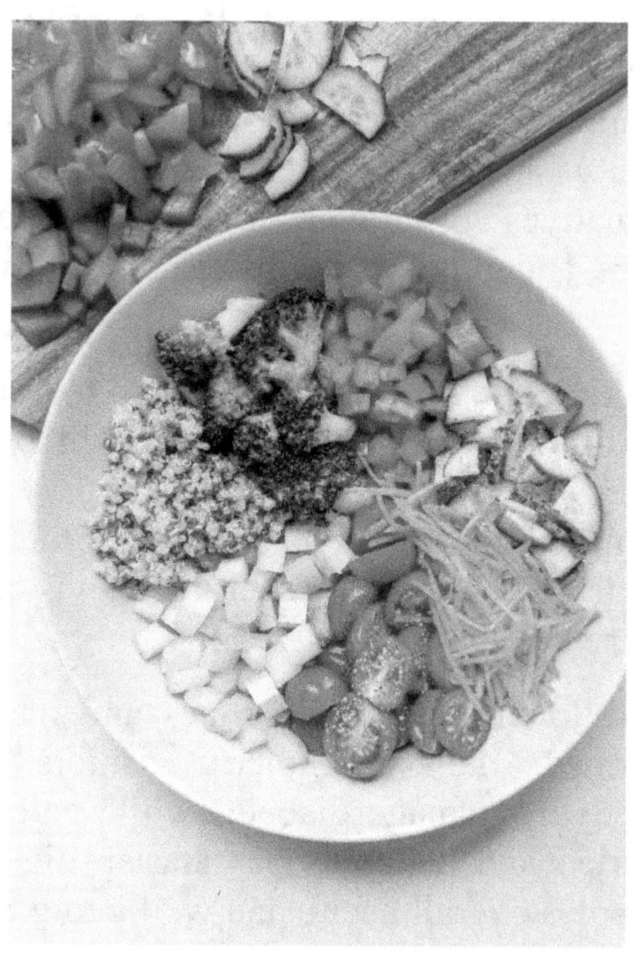

CHAPTER 4

Meal planning

Meal planning is a crucial aspect of managing diabetes on a pescatarian diet, especially for seniors. By carefully selecting and portioning out foods, seniors can maintain stable blood sugar levels, support overall health, and prevent complications associated with diabetes. Here's an explanation of meal planning for a diabetes pescatarian diet for seniors, along with its benefits for proper management:

1. Consistent Carbohydrate Distribution: Meal planning involves distributing carbohydrates evenly throughout the day to prevent sudden spikes or drops in blood sugar levels. Seniors can include complex carbohydrates like whole grains, legumes, and fruits in each meal to provide sustained energy without causing rapid fluctuations in blood glucose.

2. Balanced Macronutrient Intake: A well-planned diabetes pescatarian diet for seniors includes a balance of macronutrients—protein, carbohydrates, and fats—to promote satiety, support muscle health, and regulate blood sugar levels. By incorporating lean proteins from fish and seafood, healthy fats from nuts, seeds, and avocados, and fiber-rich carbohydrates from vegetables and whole grains, seniors can achieve a balanced meal composition.

3. Portion Control: Seniors must pay attention to portion sizes to prevent overeating and manage caloric intake effectively. Meal planning helps seniors portion out appropriate servings of different food groups, ensuring they consume adequate nutrients without consuming excessive calories or carbohydrates, which can lead to blood sugar spikes.

4. Nutrient Density: Optimizing meal plans for diabetes pescatarian diets focuses on selecting nutrient-dense foods that provide essential vitamins, minerals, and antioxidants without contributing to excessive sugar or unhealthy fats. By prioritizing whole, minimally processed foods like vegetables, fruits, whole grains, and lean proteins, seniors can maximize nutritional intake and support overall health.

5. Reduced Risk of Complications: Following a well-planned diabetes pescatarian diet reduces the risk of diabetes-related complications, such as cardiovascular disease, kidney damage, nerve damage, and vision problems. By managing blood sugar levels effectively through dietary choices, seniors can mitigate the risk of developing these complications and maintain a higher quality of life.

6. Improved Weight Management: Meal planning for diabetes pescatarian diets promotes weight management by controlling portion sizes, emphasizing nutrient-dense foods, and supporting healthy eating habits. Seniors can achieve and maintain a healthy weight, reducing the risk of obesity-related complications and improving overall metabolic health.

7. Enhanced Blood Sugar Control: Consistent meal planning ensures seniors consume a balanced mix of carbohydrates, proteins, and fats, which helps stabilize blood sugar levels throughout the day. By avoiding large fluctuations in blood glucose, seniors can reduce the risk of hyperglycemia (high blood sugar) and hypoglycemia (low blood sugar), both of which can have serious health consequences.

8. Increased Dietary Variety and Enjoyment: Meal planning allows seniors to incorporate a diverse range of foods into their diabetes pescatarian diet, enhancing flavor, texture, and culinary enjoyment. By exploring new recipes, trying different cooking techniques, and experimenting with various ingredients, seniors can maintain interest in their meals while reaping the nutritional benefits of a varied diet.

Chapter 5

RECIPES

BREAKFAST:

> **Smoked Salmon and Avocado Toast:**

Ingredients:

- 2 slices of whole grain bread

- 50g smoked salmon

- 1/2 avocado, sliced

- 1 tablespoon lemon juice

- Salt and pepper to taste

- Optional: chopped chives or dill for garnish

Preparation:

1. Toast the whole grain bread until golden brown.

2. Mash the avocado with lemon juice, salt, and pepper.

3. Spread the mashed avocado evenly on the toasted bread slices.

4. Top each slice with smoked salmon.

5. Garnish with chopped chives or dill if desired.

6. Serve immediately.

Nutritional Value:

- Calories: 300 kcal

- Protein: 15g

- Carbohydrates: 20g

- Fat: 18g

- Fiber: 7g

  ➢ **Greek Yogurt Parfait:**

  Ingredients:

- 1/2 cup Greek yogurt

- 1/4 cup fresh berries (such as strawberries, blueberries, or raspberries)

- 2 tablespoons chopped nuts (almonds, walnuts, or pecans)

- 1 tablespoon honey or maple syrup (optional)

Preparation:

1. In a serving glass or bowl, layer Greek yogurt, fresh berries, and chopped nuts.

2. Drizzle honey or maple syrup on top if desired.

3. Repeat layering if making multiple servings.

4. Serve chilled.

Nutritional Value:

- Calories: 250 kcal

- Protein: 15g

- Carbohydrates: 20g

- Fat: 12g

- Fiber: 5g

➢ **Spinach and Feta Omelette:**

Ingredients:

- 2 large eggs

- 1 cup fresh spinach leaves

- 2 tablespoons crumbled feta cheese

- Salt and pepper to taste

- 1 teaspoon olive oil

Preparation:

1. In a bowl, beat the eggs with salt and pepper.

2. Heat olive oil in a non-stick skillet over medium heat.

3. Add spinach leaves to the skillet and cook until wilted.

4. Pour beaten eggs over the spinach and let it set for a minute.

5. Sprinkle crumbled feta cheese over the omelette.

6. Fold the omelette in half and cook for another minute until fully set.

7. Slide the omelette onto a plate and serve hot.

Nutritional Value:

- Calories: 220 kcal

- Protein: 16g

- Carbohydrates: 3g

- Fat: 15g

- Fiber: 1g

➢ **Chia Seed Pudding:**

Ingredients:

- 2 tablespoons chia seeds

- 1/2 cup unsweetened almond milk

- 1/4 teaspoon vanilla extract

- 1/2 cup mixed berries for topping

- Optional: 1 tablespoon chopped nuts or shredded coconut for topping

Preparation:

1. In a bowl, mix chia seeds, almond milk, and vanilla extract.

2. Stir well to combine and let it sit for 10-15 minutes until thickened.

3. Transfer the chia seed mixture into a serving glass or bowl.

4. Top with mixed berries and optional chopped nuts or shredded coconut.

5. Serve chilled.

Nutritional Value:

- Calories: 180 kcal

- Protein: 5g

- Carbohydrates: 15g

- Fat: 10g

- Fiber: 10g

> **Veggie and Cheese Frittata:**

Ingredients:

- 4 large eggs

- 1/2 cup diced bell peppers

- 1/2 cup chopped spinach

- 1/4 cup diced tomatoes

- 1/4 cup shredded mozzarella cheese

- Salt and pepper to taste

- 1 teaspoon olive oil

Preparation:

1. Preheat the oven to 350°F (175°C).

2. In a bowl, beat the eggs with salt and pepper.

3. Heat olive oil in an oven-safe skillet over medium heat.

4. Add diced bell peppers and chopped spinach to the skillet and cook until softened.

5. Pour beaten eggs into the skillet and sprinkle diced tomatoes and shredded mozzarella cheese on top.

6. Transfer the skillet to the preheated oven and bake for 10-12 minutes until the eggs are set and the cheese is melted.

7. Remove from the oven, slice into wedges, and serve hot.

Nutritional Value:

- Calories: 280 kcal

- Protein: 20g

- Carbohydrates: 6g

- Fat: 20g

- Fiber: 2g

Ingredients:

- 1/2 cup whole wheat flour
- 1/2 teaspoon baking powder
- 1/4 teaspoon cinnamon
- 1/4 cup unsweetened almond milk
- 1 tablespoon maple syrup
- 1/2 teaspoon vanilla extract
- 1/2 cup mixed berries for topping
- Optional: Greek yogurt or chopped nuts for topping

Preparation:

1. In a bowl, whisk together whole wheat flour, baking powder, and cinnamon.

2. Stir in almond milk, maple syrup, and vanilla extract until smooth.

3. Heat a non-stick skillet or griddle over medium heat and lightly grease with cooking spray.

4. Pour 1/4 cup of the pancake batter onto the skillet and cook until bubbles form on the surface.

5. Flip the pancake and cook for another 1-2 minutes until golden brown.

6. Repeat with the remaining batter to make additional pancakes.

7. Serve pancakes topped with mixed berries and optional Greek yogurt or chopped nuts.

Nutritional Value (per pancake, without toppings):

- Calories: 100 kcal

- Protein: 3g

- Carbohydrates: 20g

- Fat: 1g

- Fiber: 3g

Ingredients:

- 1/2 block firm tofu, crumbled
- 1/2 cup diced bell peppers
- 1/4 cup diced onions
- 1/4 cup chopped mushrooms
- 1/4 cup spinach leaves
- 1/2 teaspoon turmeric powder
- Salt and pepper to taste
- 1 teaspoon olive oil

Preparation:

1. Heat olive oil in a skillet over medium heat.

2. Add diced onions and diced bell peppers to the skillet and cook until softened.

3. Stir in crumbled tofu, chopped mushrooms, and turmeric powder.

4. Cook for 5-7 minutes, stirring occasionally, until the tofu is heated through and slightly golden.

5. Add spinach leaves to the skillet and cook until wilted.

6. Season with salt and pepper to taste.

7. Serve hot.

Nutritional Value:

- Calories: 180 kcal

- Protein: 15g

- Carbohydrates: 8g

- Fat: 10g

- Fiber: 3g

Ingredients:

- 1/2 cup cooked quinoa

- 1/4 cup unsweetened almond milk

- 1/4 teaspoon cinnamon

- 1/4 cup mixed berries

- 1 tablespoon chopped nuts (such as almonds, walnuts, or pecans)

- Optional: 1 tablespoon maple syrup or honey

Preparation:

1. In a bowl, combine cooked quinoa, almond milk, and cinnamon.

2. Stir well to combine.

3. Top with mixed berries and chopped nuts.

4. Drizzle maple syrup or honey on top if desired.

5. Serve warm or cold.

Nutritional Value:

- Calories: 250 kcal

- Protein: 7g

- Carbohydrates: 35g

- Fat: 9g

- Fiber: 5g

  > **Veggie and Salmon Breakfast Wrap:**

Ingredients:

- 1 whole grain tortilla

- 50g smoked salmon

- 1/4 cup diced tomatoes

- 1/4 cup sliced cucumbers

- 2 tablespoons Greek yogurt

- Optional: chopped fresh dill or chives for garnish

Preparation:

1. Place the whole grain tortilla on a flat surface.

2. Spread Greek yogurt evenly over the tortilla.

3. Layer smoked salmon, diced tomatoes, and sliced cucumbers on top.

4. Garnish with chopped fresh dill or chives if desired.

5. Roll up the tortilla tightly.

6. Cut the wrap in half diagonally and serve.

Nutritional Value:

- Calories: 280 kcal

- Protein: 18g

- Carbohydrates: 25g

- Fat: 12g

- Fiber: 5g

Ingredients:

- 2 slices of whole grain bread
- 2 tablespoons almond butter
- 1 banana, sliced
- Optional: drizzle of honey or sprinkle of cinnamon

Preparation:

1. Toast the whole grain bread until golden brown.

2. Spread almond butter evenly on each slice of toast.

3. Arrange sliced bananas on top of the almond butter.

4. Drizzle honey or sprinkle cinnamon on top if desired.

5. Serve immediately.

Nutritional Value:

- Calories: 300 kcal

- Protein: 8g

- Carbohydrates: 35g

- Fat: 15g

- Fiber: 6g

LUNCH:

> **Mediterranean Chickpea Salad:**

Ingredients:

- 1 cup cooked chickpeas

- 1/2 cup cherry tomatoes, halved

- 1/4 cup diced cucumber

- 1/4 cup diced red onion

- 2 tablespoons chopped fresh parsley

- 1 tablespoon extra virgin olive oil

- 1 tablespoon lemon juice

- Salt and pepper to taste

Preparation:

1. In a large bowl, combine cooked chickpeas, cherry tomatoes, diced cucumber, diced red onion, and chopped fresh parsley.

2. Drizzle extra virgin olive oil and lemon juice over the salad.

3. Season with salt and pepper to taste.

4. Toss gently to combine.

5. Serve chilled or at room temperature.

Nutritional Value:

- Calories: 250 kcal

- Protein: 10g

- Carbohydrates: 30g

- Fat: 10g

- Fiber: 8g

Ingredients:

- 1 zucchini, cut into chunks
- 1 bell pepper, cut into chunks
- 1 red onion, cut into chunks
- 8 cherry tomatoes
- 100g halloumi cheese, cut into cubes
- 1 tablespoon olive oil
- 1 tablespoon balsamic vinegar
- Salt and pepper to taste

Preparation:

1. Preheat the grill or grill pan over medium-high heat.
2. Thread zucchini, bell pepper, red onion, cherry tomatoes, and halloumi cheese onto skewers.

3. In a small bowl, whisk together olive oil and balsamic vinegar.

4. Brush the skewers with the olive oil and balsamic vinegar mixture.

5. Season with salt and pepper to taste.

6. Grill the skewers for 8-10 minutes, turning occasionally, until the vegetables are tender and the halloumi is lightly browned.

7. Serve hot.

Nutritional Value:

- Calories: 280 kcal

- Protein: 15g

- Carbohydrates: 15g

- Fat: 18g

- Fiber: 3g

Ingredients:

- 1 can (5 oz) tuna, drained
- 1/4 cup diced celery
- 1/4 cup diced red bell pepper
- 2 tablespoons Greek yogurt
- 1 tablespoon lemon juice
- 1 teaspoon Dijon mustard
- Salt and pepper to taste
- 4 large lettuce leaves (such as romaine or butter lettuce)

Preparation:

1. In a bowl, combine drained tuna, diced celery, diced red bell pepper, Greek yogurt, lemon juice, and Dijon mustard.

2. Season with salt and pepper to taste.

3. Mix well to combine.

4. Divide the tuna salad evenly among the lettuce leaves.

5. Roll up the lettuce leaves to form wraps.

6. Serve immediately.

Nutritional Value:

- Calories: 200 kcal

- Protein: 20g

- Carbohydrates: 5g

- Fat: 10g

- Fiber: 2g

> **Quinoa and Black Bean Stuffed Peppers:**

Ingredients:

- 2 large bell peppers, halved and seeds removed

- 1 cup cooked quinoa

- 1 cup cooked black beans

- 1/2 cup diced tomatoes

- 1/4 cup diced red onion

- 1/4 cup chopped cilantro

- 1 teaspoon ground cumin

- 1/2 teaspoon chili powder

- Salt and pepper to taste

- Optional: shredded cheese for topping

Preparation:

1. Preheat the oven to 375°F (190°C).

2. In a large bowl, combine cooked quinoa, cooked black beans,

   diced tomatoes, diced red onion, chopped cilantro, ground cumin, chili powder, salt, and pepper.

3. Mix well to combine.

4. Stuff each bell pepper half with the quinoa and black bean mixture.

5. Place the stuffed peppers in a baking dish.

6. If using, sprinkle shredded cheese on top of the stuffed peppers.

7. Cover the baking dish with aluminum foil and bake for 25-30 minutes until the peppers are tender.

8. Remove the foil and bake for an additional 5 minutes until the cheese is melted and bubbly.

9. Serve hot.

Nutritional Value:

- Calories: 300 kcal

- Protein: 15g

- Carbohydrates: 45g

- Fat: 5g

- Fiber: 10g

Ingredients:

- 2 salmon fillets
- 1 bunch asparagus, trimmed
- 2 tablespoons olive oil
- 1 tablespoon lemon juice
- 2 cloves garlic, minced
- Salt and pepper to taste
- Optional: fresh herbs for garnish (such as dill or parsley)

Preparation:

1. Preheat the oven to 400°F (200°C).
2. Place each salmon fillet on a piece of aluminum foil.
3. Arrange asparagus around the salmon fillets.

4. In a small bowl, whisk together olive oil, lemon juice, minced garlic, salt, and pepper.

5. Drizzle the olive oil mixture over the salmon and asparagus.

6. Fold the aluminum foil to create sealed packets.

7. Place the foil packets on a baking sheet and bake for 15-20 minutes until the salmon is cooked through and the asparagus is tender.

8. Carefully open the foil packets and transfer the salmon and asparagus to plates.

9. Garnish with fresh herbs if desired.

10.   Serve hot.

Nutritional Value:

- Calories: 350 kcal

- Protein: 30g

- Carbohydrates: 8g

- Fat: 20g

- Fiber: 4g

> **Lentil and Vegetable Soup:**

Ingredients:

- 1 cup dry green lentils, rinsed

- 4 cups vegetable broth

- 1 cup diced carrots

- 1 cup diced celery

- 1 cup diced onion

- 2 cloves garlic, minced

- 1 teaspoon ground cumin

- 1/2 teaspoon smoked paprika

- Salt and pepper to taste

- 2 tablespoons chopped fresh parsley

Preparation:

1. In a large pot, combine dry green lentils, vegetable broth, diced carrots, diced celery, diced onion, minced garlic, ground cumin, smoked paprika, salt, and pepper.

2. Bring the soup to a boil over medium-high heat.

3. Reduce the heat to low, cover, and simmer for 20-25 minutes until the lentils and vegetables are tender.

4. Stir in chopped fresh parsley.

5. Adjust seasoning with additional salt and pepper if needed.

6. Serve hot.

Nutritional Value:

- Calories: 250 kcal

- Protein: 15g

- Carbohydrates: 40g

- Fat: 2g

- Fiber: 15g

Ingredients:

- 1 cup cooked quinoa

- 1/2 cup diced cucumber

- 1/2 cup cherry tomatoes, halved

- 1/4 cup diced red onion

- 1/4 cup crumbled feta cheese

- 2 tablespoons chopped Kalamata olives

- 1 tablespoon extra virgin olive oil

- 1 tablespoon red wine vinegar

- Salt and pepper to taste

- Optional: chopped fresh parsley for garnish

Preparation:

1. In a large bowl, combine cooked quinoa, diced cucumber, cherry tomatoes, diced red onion, crumbled feta cheese, and chopped Kalamata olives.

2. Drizzle extra virgin olive oil and red wine vinegar over the salad.

3. Season with salt and pepper to taste.

4. Toss gently to combine.

5. Garnish with chopped fresh parsley if desired.

6. Serve chilled or at room temperature.

Nutritional Value:

- Calories: 280 kcal

- Protein: 10g

- Carbohydrates: 30g

- Fat: 15g

- Fiber: 5g

➢ **Stuffed Portobello Mushrooms with Spinach and Feta:**

Ingredients:

- 4 large portobello mushrooms, stems removed

- 2 cups chopped spinach

- 1/4 cup diced red onion

- 1/4 cup crumbled feta cheese

- 2 cloves garlic, minced

- 1 tablespoon olive oil

- Salt and pepper to taste

Preparation:

1. Preheat the oven to 375°F (190°C).

2. Place portobello mushrooms on a baking sheet lined with parchment paper.

3. In a skillet, heat olive oil over medium heat.

4. Add minced garlic and diced red onion to the skillet and cook until softened.

5. Add chopped spinach to the skillet and cook until wilted.

6. Remove from heat and stir in crumbled feta cheese.

7. Season with salt and pepper to taste.

8. Spoon the spinach and feta mixture into the cavity of each portobello mushroom.

9. Bake for 15-20 minutes until the mushrooms are tender and the filling is heated through.

10. Serve hot.

Nutritional Value:

- Calories: 200 kcal

- Protein: 10g

- Carbohydrates: 15g

- Fat: 10g

- Fiber: 5g

➤ **Avocado and Chickpea Salad Wraps:**

Ingredients:

- 1 ripe avocado, mashed

- 1 can (15 oz) chickpeas, drained and rinsed

- 1/4 cup diced red bell pepper

- 1/4 cup diced red onion

- 2 tablespoons chopped cilantro

- 1 tablespoon lime juice

- Salt and pepper to taste

- 4 large whole grain tortillas

Preparation:

1. In a bowl, combine mashed avocado, chickpeas, diced red bell pepper, diced red onion, chopped cilantro, lime juice, salt, and pepper.

2. Mix well to combine, mashing some of the chickpeas slightly.

3. Divide the avocado and chickpea mixture evenly among the tortillas.

4. Roll up the tortillas to form wraps.

5. Serve immediately or wrap in foil for later.

Nutritional Value:

- Calories: 300 kcal

- Protein: 10g

- Carbohydrates: 40g

- Fat: 12g

- Fiber: 10g

Ingredients:

- 1/2 lb shrimp, peeled and deveined
- 2 cups mixed vegetables (such as bell peppers, broccoli, carrots, snap peas)
- 2 cloves garlic, minced
- 1 tablespoon grated ginger
- 2 tablespoons low-sodium soy sauce
- 1 tablespoon hoisin sauce
- 1 teaspoon sesame oil
- 1 tablespoon olive oil
- Optional: sliced green onions and sesame seeds for garnish

Preparation:

1. In a bowl, combine shrimp with minced garlic, grated ginger, low-sodium soy sauce, and hoisin sauce. Let marinate for 10-15 minutes.

2. Heat olive oil in a skillet or wok over medium-high heat.

3. Add mixed vegetables to the skillet and stir-fry for 3-4 minutes until slightly tender.

4. Push the vegetables to one side of the skillet and add marinated shrimp to the other side.

5. Cook shrimp for 2-3 minutes on each side until pink and cooked through.

6. Stir in sesame oil and toss everything together.

7. Remove from heat and garnish with sliced green onions and sesame seeds if desired.

8. Serve hot over cooked quinoa or brown rice if desired.

Nutritional Value:

- Calories: 250 kcal

- Protein: 20g

- Carbohydrates: 15g

- Fat: 10g

- Fiber: 5g

➢ Baked Lemon Garlic Salmon:

Ingredients:

- 2 salmon fillets

- 2 cloves garlic, minced

- 1 tablespoon lemon juice

- 1 teaspoon lemon zest

- 1 tablespoon olive oil

- Salt and pepper to taste

- Fresh herbs for garnish (such as parsley or dill)

Preparation:

1. Preheat the oven to 375°F (190°C).

2. In a small bowl, combine minced garlic, lemon juice, lemon zest, olive oil, salt, and pepper.

3. Place salmon fillets on a baking sheet lined with parchment paper.

4. Brush the lemon garlic mixture over the salmon fillets.

5. Bake for 12-15 minutes until the salmon is cooked through and flakes easily with a fork.

6. Garnish with fresh herbs before serving.

Nutritional Value:

- Calories: 300 kcal

- Protein: 25g

- Carbohydrates: 1g

- Fat: 20g

- Fiber: 0g

➢ **Quinoa Stuffed Bell Peppers:**

Ingredients:

- 4 large bell peppers, halved and seeds removed

- 1 cup cooked quinoa

- 1 cup black beans, drained and rinsed

- 1 cup diced tomatoes

- 1/2 cup diced red onion

- 1/2 cup corn kernels

- 1 teaspoon ground cumin

- 1/2 teaspoon chili powder

- Salt and pepper to taste

- Optional: shredded cheese for topping

Preparation:

1. Preheat the oven to 375°F (190°C).

2. In a large bowl, combine cooked quinoa, black beans, diced tomatoes,

diced red onion, corn kernels, ground cumin, chili powder, salt, and pepper.

3. Spoon the quinoa mixture into each bell pepper half.

4. Place stuffed bell peppers in a baking dish.

5. If using, sprinkle shredded cheese on top of the stuffed peppers.

6. Cover the baking dish with aluminum foil and bake for 25-30 minutes until the peppers are tender.

7. Remove the foil and bake for an additional 5 minutes until the cheese is melted and bubbly.

8. Serve hot.

Nutritional Value:

- Calories: 280 kcal

- Protein: 15g

- Carbohydrates: 40g

- Fat: 5g

- Fiber: 10g

➢ **Garlic Shrimp and Broccoli Stir-Fry:**

Ingredients:

- 1/2 lb shrimp, peeled and deveined

- 2 cups broccoli florets

- 2 cloves garlic, minced

- 1 tablespoon low-sodium soy sauce

- 1 teaspoon sesame oil

- 1 tablespoon olive oil

- Salt and pepper to taste

Preparation:

1. Heat olive oil in a skillet or wok over medium-high heat.

2. Add minced garlic to the skillet and cook for 1 minute until fragrant.

3. Add shrimp to the skillet and cook for 2-3 minutes on each side until pink and cooked through.

4. Remove shrimp from the skillet and set aside.

5. In the same skillet, add broccoli florets and cook for 3-4 minutes until tender-crisp.

6. Return cooked shrimp to the skillet.

7. Drizzle low-sodium soy sauce and sesame oil over the shrimp and broccoli.

8. Toss everything together until well combined.

9. Season with salt and pepper to taste.

10. Serve hot.

Nutritional Value:

- Calories: 250 kcal

- Protein: 20g

- Carbohydrates: 10g

- Fat: 10g

- Fiber: 4g

➢ **Mediterranean Baked Cod:**

Ingredients:

- 2 cod fillets

- 1/4 cup diced tomatoes

- 2 tablespoons chopped Kalamata olives

- 2 tablespoons chopped fresh parsley

- 1 tablespoon olive oil

- 1 tablespoon lemon juice

- 1 clove garlic, minced

- Salt and pepper to taste

Preparation:

1. Preheat the oven to 375°F (190°C).

2. Place cod fillets on a baking sheet lined with parchment paper.

3. In a small bowl, combine diced tomatoes, chopped Kalamata olives, chopped fresh parsley, olive oil, lemon juice, minced garlic, salt, and pepper.

4. Spoon the tomato olive mixture over the cod fillets.

5. Bake for 12-15 minutes until the cod is cooked through and flakes easily with a fork.

6. Serve hot.

Nutritional Value:

- Calories: 200 kcal

- Protein: 25g

- Carbohydrates: 3g

- Fat: 8g

- Fiber: 1g

Ingredients:

- 2 tilapia fillets
- 1 tablespoon olive oil
- 1 tablespoon lemon juice
- 1 teaspoon lemon zest
- 1 teaspoon dried thyme
- 1 teaspoon dried oregano
- Salt and pepper to taste

Preparation:

1. Preheat the oven to 375°F (190°C).

2. Place tilapia fillets on a baking sheet lined with parchment paper.

3. In a small bowl, whisk together olive oil, lemon juice, lemon zest, dried thyme, dried oregano, salt, and pepper.

4. Brush the lemon herb mixture over the tilapia fillets.

5. Bake for 10-12 minutes until the tilapia is cooked through and flakes easily with a fork.

6. Serve hot.

Nutritional Value:

- Calories: 180 kcal

- Protein: 20g

- Carbohydrates: 1g

- Fat: 10g

- Fiber: 0g

> Vegetarian Lentil Soup:

Ingredients:

- 1 cup dry green lentils, rinsed

- 4 cups vegetable broth

- 1 cup diced carrots

- 1 cup diced celery

- 1 cup diced onion

- 2 cloves garlic, minced

- 1 teaspoon ground cumin

- 1/2 teaspoon smoked paprika

- Salt and pepper to taste

- 2 tablespoons chopped fresh parsley

Preparation:

1. In a large pot, combine dry green lentils, vegetable broth, diced carrots, diced celery, diced onion, minced garlic, ground cumin, smoked paprika, salt, and pepper.

2. Bring the soup to a boil over medium-high heat.

3. Reduce the heat to low, cover, and simmer for 20-25 minutes until the lentils and vegetables are tender.

4. Stir in chopped fresh parsley.

5. Adjust seasoning with additional salt and pepper if needed.

6. Serve hot.

Nutritional Value:

- Calories: 250 kcal

- Protein: 15g

- Carbohydrates: 40g

- Fat: 2g

- Fiber: 15g

➤ **Spaghetti Squash with Tomato Basil Sauce:**

Ingredients:

- 1 medium spaghetti squash

- 1 cup tomato basil sauce (store-bought or homemade)

- 2 tablespoons grated Parmesan cheese

- Fresh basil leaves for garnish

- Salt and pepper to taste

Preparation:

1. Preheat the oven to 400°F (200°C).

2. Cut the spaghetti squash in half lengthwise and scoop out the seeds.

3. Place the squash halves cut side down on a baking sheet lined with parchment paper.

4. Bake for 40-45 minutes until the squash is tender.

5. Use a fork to scrape the flesh of the squash into spaghetti-like strands.

6. Heat tomato basil sauce in a saucepan over medium heat until warmed through.

7. Divide the spaghetti squash strands among serving plates.

8. Spoon tomato basil sauce over the spaghetti squash.

9. Sprinkle grated Parmesan cheese on top.

10. Garnish with fresh basil leaves.

11. Serve hot.

Nutritional Value:

- Calories: 200 kcal

- Protein: 5g

- Carbohydrates: 30g

- Fat: 8g

- Fiber: 8g

> **Pesto Zucchini Noodles with Cherry Tomatoes:**

Ingredients:

- 2 medium zucchinis, spiralized into noodles

- 1 cup cherry tomatoes, halved

- 2 tablespoons pesto sauce (store-bought or homemade)

- 2 tablespoons grated Parmesan cheese

- Salt and pepper to taste

Preparation:

1. Heat a large skillet over medium heat.

2. Add spiralized zucchini noodles to the skillet and cook for 2-3 minutes until just tender.

3. Add cherry tomatoes to the skillet and cook for another 1-2 minutes until heated through.

4. Stir in pesto sauce until well combined.

5. Season with salt and pepper to taste.

6. Remove from heat and sprinkle grated Parmesan cheese on top.

7. Serve immediately.

Nutritional Value:

- Calories: 150 kcal

- Protein: 5g

- Carbohydrates: 10g

- Fat: 10g

- Fiber: 3g

> ## Stuffed Eggplant with Quinoa and Feta:

Ingredients:

- 2 medium eggplants

- 1 cup cooked quinoa

- 1/2 cup crumbled feta cheese

- 1/4 cup diced tomatoes

- 2 tablespoons chopped fresh parsley

- 1 clove garlic, minced

- 1 tablespoon olive oil

- Salt and pepper to taste

Preparation:

1. Preheat the oven to 375°F (190°C).

2. Cut the eggplants in half lengthwise and scoop out the flesh, leaving about a 1/2-inch shell.

3. Chop the eggplant flesh and set aside.

4. In a skillet, heat olive oil over medium heat.

5. Add minced garlic to the skillet and cook for 1 minute until fragrant.

6. Add chopped eggplant flesh to the skillet and cook for 5-7 minutes until softened.

7. Remove from heat and stir in cooked quinoa, crumbled feta cheese, diced tomatoes, chopped fresh parsley, salt, and pepper.

8. Stuff the eggplant shells with the quinoa mixture.

9. Place stuffed eggplants on a baking sheet lined with parchment paper.

10.   Bake for 25-30 minutes until the eggplants are tender and the filling is heated through.

11.   Serve hot.

Nutritional Value:

- Calories: 250 kcal

- Protein: 10g

- Carbohydrates: 30g

- Fat: 10g

- Fiber: 8g

> ## Coconut Curry Shrimp with Vegetables:

Ingredients:

- 1/2 lb shrimp, peeled and deveined

- 2 cups mixed vegetables (such as bell peppers, broccoli, carrots, snap peas)

- 1 can (13.5 oz) coconut milk

- 2 tablespoons red curry paste

- 1 tablespoon fish sauce

- 1 tablespoon lime juice

- 1 tablespoon olive oil

- Optional: chopped fresh cilantro for garnish

Preparation:

1. Heat olive oil in a large skillet or wok over medium-high heat.

2. Add mixed vegetables to the skillet and stir-fry for 3-4 minutes until slightly tender.

3. Push the vegetables to one side of the skillet and add shrimp to the other side.

4. Cook shrimp for 2-3 minutes on each side until pink and cooked through.

5. In a small bowl, whisk together coconut milk, red curry paste, fish sauce, and lime juice.

6. Pour the coconut curry mixture over the shrimp and vegetables in the skillet.

7. Stir everything together until well combined.

8. Simmer for 2-3 minutes until heated through.

9. Garnish with chopped fresh cilantro if desired.

10.   Serve hot over cooked brown rice or quinoa if desired.

Nutritional Value:

- Calories: 300 kcal

- Protein: 20g

- Carbohydrates: 15g

- Fat: 20g

- Fiber: 4g

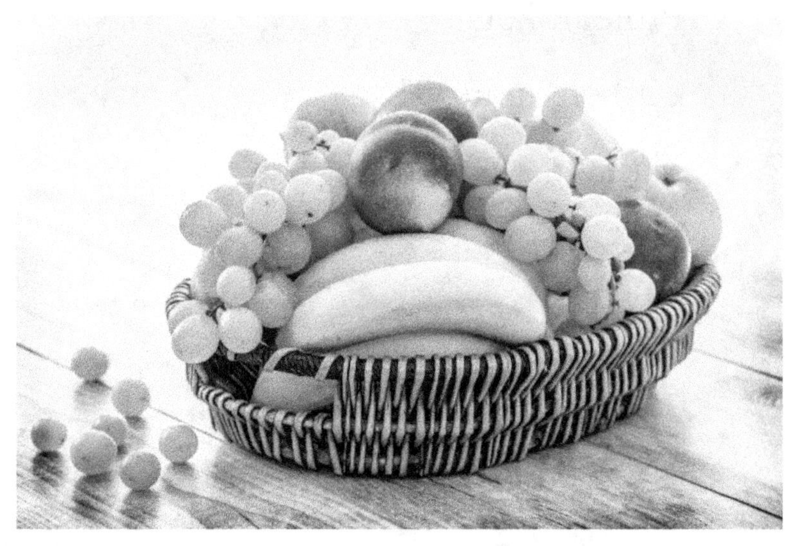

In this diabetic pescatarian diet cookbook serves as a comprehensive guide to maintaining a healthy lifestyle while managing diabetes. By focusing on nutritious and flavorful anti-inflammatory recipes, seniors can naturally combat inflammation and enhance their overall health. With a wide variety of breakfast, lunch, and dinner options, each recipe provides essential nutrients without compromising on taste. The emphasis on pescatarian ingredients ensures a rich source of protein and healthy fats, while also promoting heart health and weight management. By following this cookbook, seniors can enjoy delicious meals that not only support their dietary needs but also contribute to better blood sugar control and overall well-being. Remember, embracing this diet is not just about managing diabetes, but also about embracing a fulfilling and vibrant life.

With dedication and commitment, adopting and adapting to this diet can lead to a happier, healthier, and more energetic lifestyle. Start your journey towards improved health today and savor the delicious flavors of these diabetes-friendly pescatarian recipes.

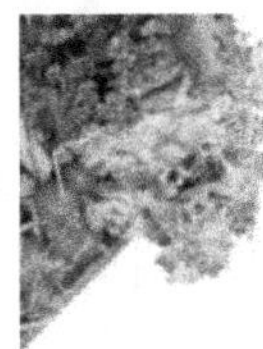

WEEKLY MEAL PLANNER

MONDAY	BREAKFAST	
	LUNCH	
	DINNER	
TUESDAY	BREAKFAST	
	LUNCH	
	DINNER	
WEDNESDAY	BREAKFAST	
	LUNCH	
	DINNER	
THURSDAY	BREAKFAST	
	LUNCH	
	DINNER	
FRIDAY	BREAKFAST	
	LUNCH	
	DINNER	
SARTURDAY	BREAKFAST	
	LUNCH	
	DINNER	
SUNDAY	BREAKFAST	
	LUNCH	
	DINNER	

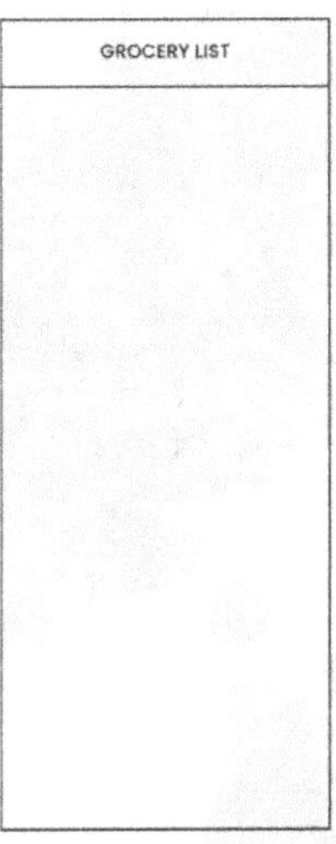

GROCERY LIST

SNACKS

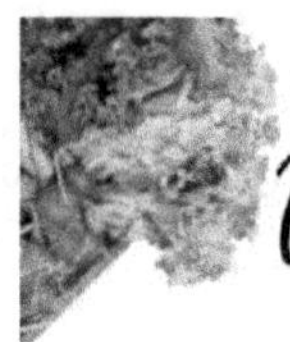

WEEKLY MEAL PLANNER

			GROCERY LIST
MONDAY	BREAKFAST		
	LUNCH		
	DINNER		
TUESDAY	BREAKFAST		
	LUNCH		
	DINNER		
WEDNESDAY	BREAKFAST		
	LUNCH		
	DINNER		
THURSDAY	BREAKFAST		
	LUNCH		
	DINNER		
FRIDAY	BREAKFAST		SNACKS
	LUNCH		
	DINNER		
SARTURDAY	BREAKFAST		
	LUNCH		
	DINNER		
SUNDAY	BREAKFAST		
	LUNCH		
	DINNER		

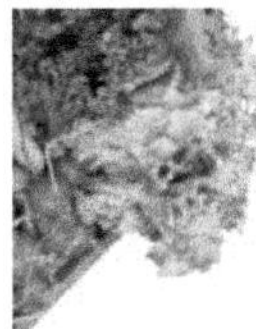

WEEKLY MEAL PLANNER

MONDAY	BREAKFAST	
	LUNCH	
	DINNER	
TUESDAY	BREAKFAST	
	LUNCH	
	DINNER	
WEDNESDAY	BREAKFAST	
	LUNCH	
	DINNER	
THURSDAY	BREAKFAST	
	LUNCH	
	DINNER	
FRIDAY	BREAKFAST	
	LUNCH	
	DINNER	
SARTURDAY	BREAKFAST	
	LUNCH	
	DINNER	
SUNDAY	BREAKFAST	
	LUNCH	
	DINNER	

GROCERY LIST

SNACKS

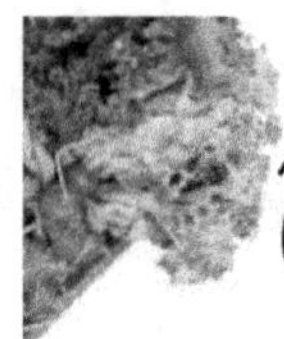

WEEKLY MEAL PLANNER

MONDAY	BREAKFAST	
	LUNCH	
	DINNER	
TUESDAY	BREAKFAST	
	LUNCH	
	DINNER	
WEDNESDAY	BREAKFAST	
	LUNCH	
	DINNER	
THURSDAY	BREAKFAST	
	LUNCH	
	DINNER	
FRIDAY	BREAKFAST	
	LUNCH	
	DINNER	
SARTURDAY	BREAKFAST	
	LUNCH	
	DINNER	
SUNDAY	BREAKFAST	
	LUNCH	
	DINNER	

GROCERY LIST

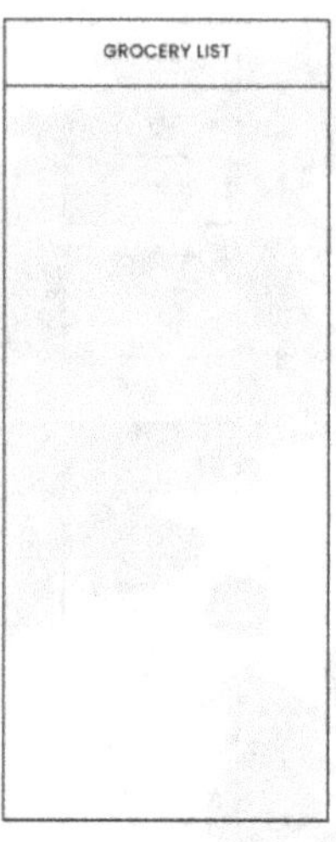

SNACKS

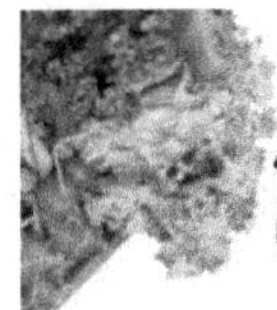

WEEKLY MEAL PLANNER

MONDAY	BREAKFAST	
	LUNCH	
	DINNER	
TUESDAY	BREAKFAST	
	LUNCH	
	DINNER	
WEDNESDAY	BREAKFAST	
	LUNCH	
	DINNER	
THURSDAY	BREAKFAST	
	LUNCH	
	DINNER	
FRIDAY	BREAKFAST	
	LUNCH	
	DINNER	
SARTURDAY	BREAKFAST	
	LUNCH	
	DINNER	
SUNDAY	BREAKFAST	
	LUNCH	
	DINNER	

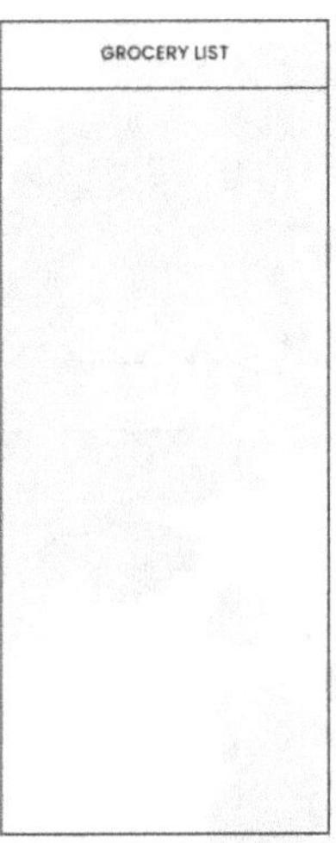

GROCERY LIST

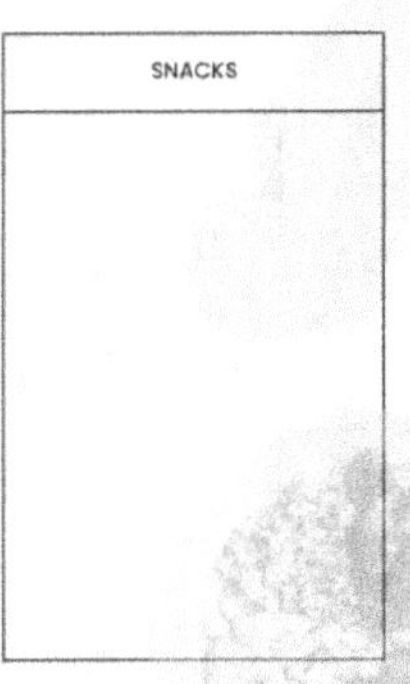

SNACKS

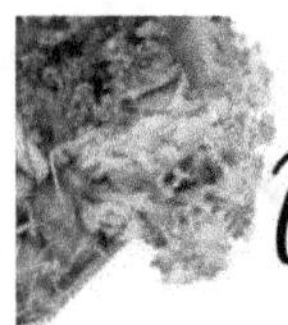

WEEKLY MEAL PLANNER

	MONDAY	
	BREAKFAST	
	LUNCH	
	DINNER	

	TUESDAY	
	BREAKFAST	
	LUNCH	
	DINNER	

	WEDNESDAY	
	BREAKFAST	
	LUNCH	
	DINNER	

	THURSDAY	
	BREAKFAST	
	LUNCH	
	DINNER	

	FRIDAY	
	BREAKFAST	
	LUNCH	
	DINNER	

	SARTURDAY	
	BREAKFAST	
	LUNCH	
	DINNER	

	SUNDAY	
	BREAKFAST	
	LUNCH	
	DINNER	

GROCERY LIST

SNACKS

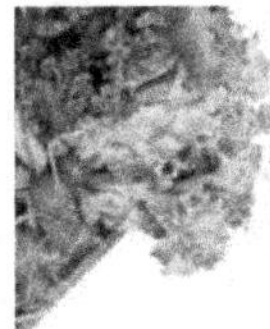

WEEKLY MEAL PLANNER

MONDAY	BREAKFAST	
	LUNCH	
	DINNER	
TUESDAY	BREAKFAST	
	LUNCH	
	DINNER	
WEDNESDAY	BREAKFAST	
	LUNCH	
	DINNER	
THURSDAY	BREAKFAST	
	LUNCH	
	DINNER	
FRIDAY	BREAKFAST	
	LUNCH	
	DINNER	
SARTURDAY	BREAKFAST	
	LUNCH	
	DINNER	
SUNDAY	BREAKFAST	
	LUNCH	
	DINNER	

GROCERY LIST

SNACKS

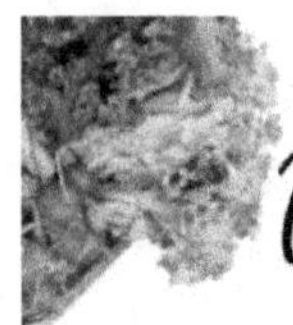

WEEKLY MEAL PLANNER

MONDAY	BREAKFAST	
	LUNCH	
	DINNER	
TUESDAY	BREAKFAST	
	LUNCH	
	DINNER	
WEDNESDAY	BREAKFAST	
	LUNCH	
	DINNER	
THURSDAY	BREAKFAST	
	LUNCH	
	DINNER	
FRIDAY	BREAKFAST	
	LUNCH	
	DINNER	
SARTURDAY	BREAKFAST	
	LUNCH	
	DINNER	
SUNDAY	BREAKFAST	
	LUNCH	
	DINNER	

GROCERY LIST

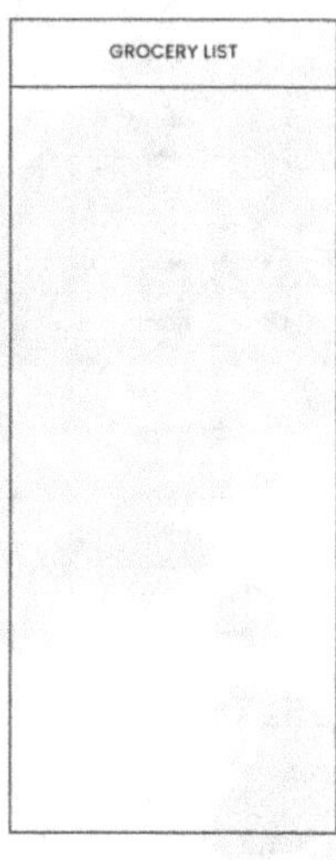

SNACKS

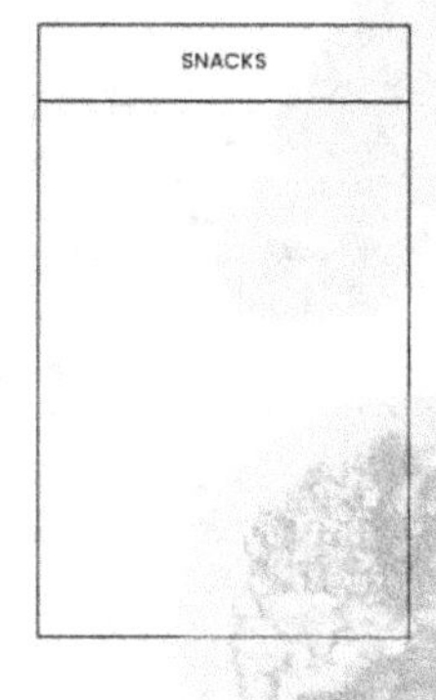

WEEKLY MEAL PLANNER

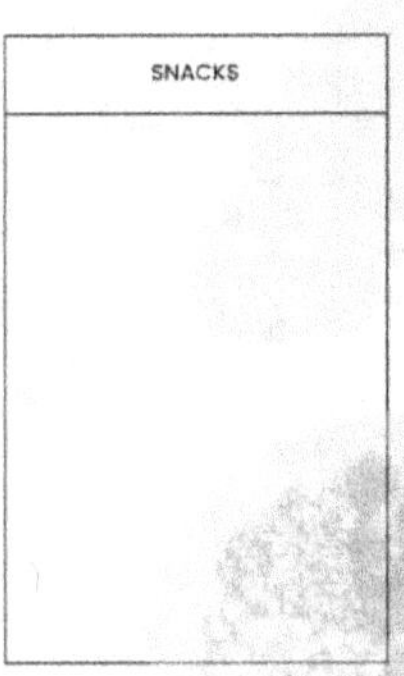

MONDAY	BREAKFAST	
	LUNCH	
	DINNER	
TUESDAY	BREAKFAST	
	LUNCH	
	DINNER	
WEDNESDAY	BREAKFAST	
	LUNCH	
	DINNER	
THURSDAY	BREAKFAST	
	LUNCH	
	DINNER	
FRIDAY	BREAKFAST	
	LUNCH	
	DINNER	
SARTURDAY	BREAKFAST	
	LUNCH	
	DINNER	
SUNDAY	BREAKFAST	
	LUNCH	
	DINNER	

GROCERY LIST

SNACKS

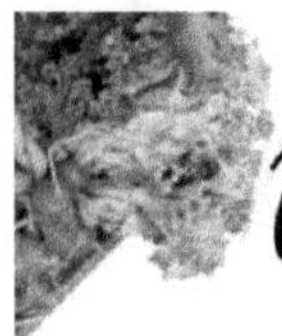

WEEKLY MEAL PLANNER

MONDAY	BREAKFAST	
	LUNCH	
	DINNER	
TUESDAY	BREAKFAST	
	LUNCH	
	DINNER	
WEDNESDAY	BREAKFAST	
	LUNCH	
	DINNER	
THURSDAY	BREAKFAST	
	LUNCH	
	DINNER	
FRIDAY	BREAKFAST	
	LUNCH	
	DINNER	
SARTURDAY	BREAKFAST	
	LUNCH	
	DINNER	
SUNDAY	BREAKFAST	
	LUNCH	
	DINNER	

GROCERY LIST

SNACKS

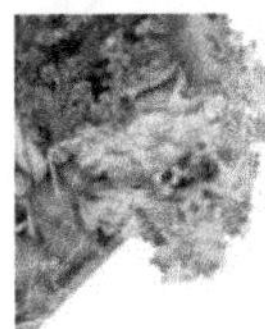

WEEKLY MEAL PLANNER

				GROCERY LIST
MONDAY	BREAKFAST			
	LUNCH			
	DINNER			
TUESDAY	BREAKFAST			
	LUNCH			
	DINNER			
WEDNESDAY	BREAKFAST			
	LUNCH			
	DINNER			
THURSDAY	BREAKFAST			
	LUNCH			
	DINNER			
FRIDAY	BREAKFAST			
	LUNCH			SNACKS
	DINNER			
SARTURDAY	BREAKFAST			
	LUNCH			
	DINNER			
SUNDAY	BREAKFAST			
	LUNCH			
	DINNER			

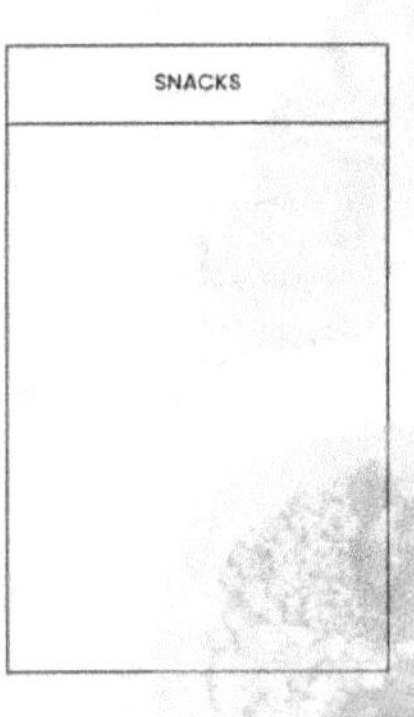

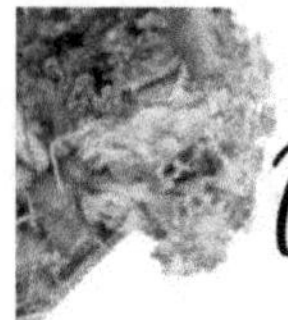

WEEKLY MEAL PLANNER

MONDAY	BREAKFAST	
	LUNCH	
	DINNER	
TUESDAY	BREAKFAST	
	LUNCH	
	DINNER	
WEDNESDAY	BREAKFAST	
	LUNCH	
	DINNER	
THURSDAY	BREAKFAST	
	LUNCH	
	DINNER	
FRIDAY	BREAKFAST	
	LUNCH	
	DINNER	
SARTURDAY	BREAKFAST	
	LUNCH	
	DINNER	
SUNDAY	BREAKFAST	
	LUNCH	
	DINNER	

GROCERY LIST

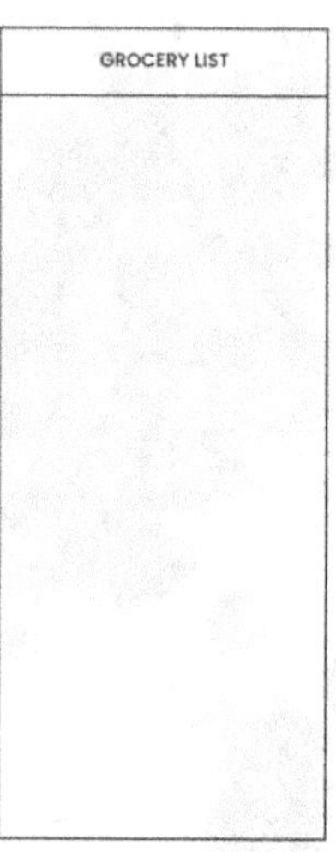

SNACKS

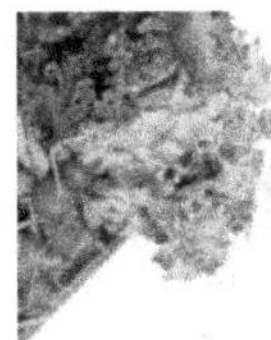

WEEKLY MEAL PLANNER

			GROCERY LIST
MONDAY	BREAKFAST		
	LUNCH		
	DINNER		
TUESDAY	BREAKFAST		
	LUNCH		
	DINNER		
WEDNESDAY	BREAKFAST		
	LUNCH		
	DINNER		
THURSDAY	BREAKFAST		
	LUNCH		
	DINNER		
FRIDAY	BREAKFAST		
	LUNCH		SNACKS
	DINNER		
SARTURDAY	BREAKFAST		
	LUNCH		
	DINNER		
SUNDAY	BREAKFAST		
	LUNCH		
	DINNER		

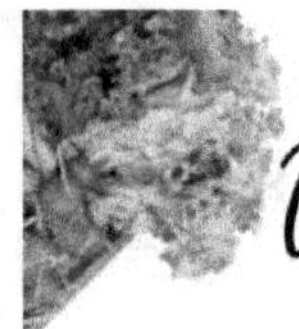

WEEKLY MEAL PLANNER

MONDAY	BREAKFAST	
	LUNCH	
	DINNER	
TUESDAY	BREAKFAST	
	LUNCH	
	DINNER	
WEDNESDAY	BREAKFAST	
	LUNCH	
	DINNER	
THURSDAY	BREAKFAST	
	LUNCH	
	DINNER	
FRIDAY	BREAKFAST	
	LUNCH	
	DINNER	
SARTURDAY	BREAKFAST	
	LUNCH	
	DINNER	
SUNDAY	BREAKFAST	
	LUNCH	
	DINNER	

GROCERY LIST

SNACKS